Transform Your Health and
Body from the Comfort of
Your Own Home

Body Revolution

Andrei Adrian

The Body Revolution

Is a movement that focuses on the idea that you can improve your health and fitness from the comfort of your own home.

This approach to wellness emphasizes the use of bodyweight exercises, mindfulness practices, and other activities that can be done at home without the need for expensive gym equipment or memberships.

The goal of the Body Revolution is to make health and wellness more accessible to people of all fitness levels, backgrounds, and budgets. By focusing on activities that can be done at home, the Body Revolution aims to help people incorporate healthy habits into their daily lives without the need for costly gym memberships or complicated workout routines.

Regular exercise is important for weight loss and overall health because it helps to burn calories and build muscle.
This can lead to a healthy body weight and a lower risk of conditions such as obesity, heart disease, and type 2 diabetes.
Exercise can also improve mental health, reduce stress, and increase energy levels.

Doing exercises at home has several benefits. It is convenient and can save time and money compared to going to a gym.
It also allows for more flexibility and control over the workout routine.

Home workouts can be tailored to individual needs and preferences, and can be done at any time and in any space that is available.

Additionally, doing exercises at home can help to reduce the risk of exposure to germs and infections that might be present in public places, such as a gym.

CHAPTER 1
Movements to do before starting the main workout

Neck rolls:

Slowly roll the head from side to side, then front to back, to loosen the neck muscles and improve range of motion.

Shoulder shrugs:

Raise the shoulders up towards the ears, then release them down, to loosen the upper back and shoulder muscles.

Arm circles:

Extend the arms out to the sides, and make small circles with the wrists, then larger circles with the shoulders, to warm up the upper body.

Torso twists:

Place the hands on the hips, and twist the torso from side to side, to loosen the spine and lower back muscles.

Hip circles:

Stand with the feet hip-width apart, and make small circles with the hips, then larger circles with the whole body, to warm up the lower body.

Ankle circles:

Stand on one foot, and make small circles with the ankle, then switch to the other foot, to warm up the lower legs and feet.

These stretches and movements can help to prepare the body for the main workout, and can reduce the risk of injuries by warming up the muscles and increasing blood flow.

It is important to start slowly and gradually increase the intensity, to avoid overstretching or straining the muscles.

CHAPTER 2
10 exercises that can be done at home to get the heart rate up and burn calories

Jumping jacks:

Start in a standing position with the feet together and the arms by the sides. Jump and spread the legs out to the sides, while raising the arms above the head. Jump back to the starting position, and repeat.

Burpees:

Start in a standing position with the feet hip-width apart. Squat down and place the hands on the floor, then kick the feet back into a plank position. Do a push-up, then quickly bring the feet back to the squat position. Stand up, and jump with the arms raised above the head. Repeat.

Running on the spot:

Start in a standing position with the feet hip-width apart. Lift the knees up, and pump the arms back and forth, to simulate running.

High knees:
Start in a standing position with the feet hip-width apart. Lift one knee up towards the chest, then quickly switch to the other knee.
Continue alternating legs, and try to lift the knees as high as possible.

Mountain climbers:
Start in a plank position with the hands under the shoulders and the feet hip-width apart. Bring one knee up towards the chest, then quickly switch to the other knee.
Continue alternating legs, and try to move quickly.

Jumping lunges:
Start in a lunge position with the left leg forward and the right leg back.
Jump up and switch legs, so the right leg is now forward and the left leg is back.
Continue alternating legs, and try to land softly.

Plank jacks:

Start in a plank position with the hands under the shoulders and the feet hip-width apart. Jump the feet out to the sides, then quickly back to the starting position. Repeat.

Side skaters:

Start in a standing position with the feet hip-width apart. Jump to the right, landing on the right foot and bringing the left foot behind. Jump to the left, landing on the left foot and bringing the right foot behind. Continue alternating sides, and try to move quickly.

Squat jumps:

Start in a standing position with the feet hip-width apart. Squat down, then quickly jump up, reaching the arms up towards the sky. Land softly, and repeat.

Stair sprints:
If you have stairs at home, sprint up
the stairs for 30 seconds, then walk back
down to recover.
Repeat for several rounds.

CHAPTER 3
Exercises that can be done at home to build muscle and increase strength

Push-ups:

Start in a plank position with the hands under the shoulders and the feet hip-width apart. Lower the body down until the chest touches the floor, then push back up to the starting position.

Squats:

Start in a standing position with the feet hip-width apart. Lower the body down as if sitting back into a chair, keeping the chest up and the weight in the heels. Push back up to the starting position.

Lunges:

Start in a standing position with the feet hip-width apart. Take a large step forward with the right foot, and lower the body down until the right thigh is parallel to the floor and the left knee is hovering above the floor.
Push back up to the starting position, and repeat on the other side.

Planks:

Start in a plank position with the hands
under the shoulders and the feet
hip-width apart.
Hold the position, keeping the body
straight and the abs engaged, for
30 seconds or more.

Sit-ups:

Start lying on the back with the knees bent
and the feet flat on the floor.
Place the hands behind the head, and lift
the upper body up towards the knees.
Lower back down, and repeat.

Dips:

Use two sturdy chairs or benches, and place
them facing each other.
Sit on the edge of one chair, and place the
hands on the edge of the other chair.
Lower the body down, then push back up,
using the triceps muscles.

Russian twists:

Start sitting on the floor with the knees bent and the feet flat on the floor.
Hold a weight or a ball in the hands, and lean back slightly.
Twist the torso to the right, then to the left, and repeat.

Glute bridges:

Start lying on the back with the knees bent and the feet flat on the floor.
Lift the hips

CHAPTER 4

Exercises that can be done at home to strengthen the abdominal and back muscles

Sit-ups:

Start lying on the back with the knees bent
and the feet flat on the floor.
Place the hands behind the head, and lift
the upper body up towards the knees.
Lower back down, and repeat.

Planks:

Start in a plank position with the hands
under the shoulders and the feet
hip-width apart.
Hold the position, keeping the body
straight and the abs engaged, for
30 seconds or more.

Glute bridges:

Start lying on the back with the knees bent
and the feet flat on the floor.
Lift the hips up towards the ceiling,
squeezing the glutes and the abs, then
lower back down.

Bicycle crunches:

Start lying on the back with the hands behind the head and the legs in the air. Bring the left elbow to the right knee, then switch sides, and continue alternating.

Mountain climbers:

Start in a plank position with the hands under the shoulders and the feet hip-width apart. Bring one knee up towards the chest, then quickly switch to the other knee. Continue alternating legs, and try to move quickly.

Scissor kicks:

Start lying on the back with the hands behind the head and the legs in the air. Cross the left leg over the right leg, then switch sides, and continue alternating.

Leg raises:

Start lying on the back with the hands under the butt and the legs straight. Lift

CHAPTER 5

Exercises that can be done at home to improve flexibility and reduce stiffness

Downward-facing dog:
Start on the hands and knees, with the wrists under the shoulders and the knees under the hips. Lift the hips up and back, and straighten the legs, forming an inverted V shape with the body.
Hold the position, and try to straighten the arms and legs as much as possible.

Forward fold:
Start standing with the feet hip-width apart. Hinge at the hips, and fold the upper body down towards the legs, keeping the knees soft and the back straight.
Hold the position, and try to touch the hands to the ground or the feet.

Low lunge:
Start standing with the feet hip-width apart. Step the right foot forward, and lower the lef knee down to the ground. Place the hands or the right thigh, and straighten the right leg. Hold the position, and try to push the hips forward and the chest up.

Pigeon pose:

Start on the hands and knees, with the wrists under the shoulders and the knees under the hips. Bring the right foot forward and place it near the left hand, then lower the right knee down and straighten the left leg behind.
Place the hands on the ground or on blocks, and hold the position, trying to push the hips back and down.

Child's pose:

Start on the hands and knees, with the wrists under the shoulders and the knees under the hips. Sit back on the heels, and fold the upper body down towards the ground, stretching the arms out in front or by the sides.
Hold the position, and try to relax the whole body.

Cat-cow stretch:

Start on the hands and knees, with the wrists under the shoulders and the knees under the hips. Round the spine up towards the ceiling, then arch the back down towards the ground, moving with the breath.
Repeat several times, and try to move smoothly and slowly.

Chest opener:

Start standing with the feet hip-width apart. Interlace the fingers behind the back, and lift the arms up towards the sky, stretching the chest and the shoulders. Hold the position, and try to push the arms back and the chest forward.

Hamstring stretch:

Start sitting on the ground with the legs straight in front. Reach the hands towards the feet, and try to touch the toes or the shins.
Hold the position, and try to keep the back straight and the legs engaged.

Shoulder stretch:
Start standing with the feet hip-width apart.
Reach the right arm across the chest, and
grab the left elbow with the right hand.
Hold the position, and try to pull the elbow
towards the chest, feeling a stretch in the
right shoulder.
Repeat on the other side.

Foam rolling:
Use a foam roller to massage

CHAPTER 6

Some simple stretches and movements to do after the workout

These stretches and movements can help to cool down the body after the workout, and can reduce the risk of soreness by releasing tension and restoring flexibility.

Chest and shoulder stretch:

Start standing with the feet hip-width apart. Reach the right arm across the chest, and grab the left elbow with the right hand. Hold the position, and try to pull the elbow towards the chest, feeling a stretch in the right shoulder.
Repeat on the other side.

Hamstring stretch:

Start sitting on the ground with the legs straight in front. Reach the hands towards the feet, and try to touch the toes or the shins. Hold the position, and try to keep the back straight and the legs engaged.

Quadriceps stretch:

Start standing with the feet hip-width apart. Hold onto a wall or a chair for balance, and grab the right ankle with the right hand. Pull the heel towards the butt, feeling a stretch in the front of the right thigh.
Repeat on the other side.

Groin stretch:

Start sitting on the ground with the legs spread out to the sides in a diamond shape. Reach the hands towards the feet, and try to touch the toes or the shins.
Hold the position, and try to keep the back straight and the legs engaged.

Calf stretch:

Start standing with the feet hip-width apart. Step the right foot back, and press the heel down towards the ground, feeling a stretch in the calf muscles.
Repeat on the other side.

Neck stretch:

Start sitting or standing with the feet hip-width apart. Tilt the head to the right, then to the left, and finally down towards the chest, feeling a stretch in the neck muscles.

CHAPTER 7
Benefits of regular exercise

Burning calories:
Exercise helps to burn calories and increase metabolism, which can lead to weight loss and a healthy body weight.

Building muscle:
Exercise can help to build and strengthen muscles, which can improve strength and physical performance.

Improving overall health:
Exercise has numerous health benefits, such as reducing the risk of chronic diseases, such as heart disease, stroke, and type 2 diabetes. Exercise can also improve mental health, reduce stress, and increase energy levels.

Enhancing cognitive function:
Exercise has been shown to improve brain function and cognitive abilities, such as memory, concentration, and decision making.

Improving sleep:

Exercise can help to improve sleep quality, and can make it easier to fall asleep and stay asleep.

Boosting mood:

Exercise can help to boost mood and reduce symptoms of depression and anxiety. It can also increase self-esteem and body confidence.

Overall, regular exercise can have a positive impact on overall health and well-being. It is an important part of a healthy lifestyle, and can help to improve physical, mental, and emotional health.

CHAPTER 8
Tips for maintaining a regular exercise routine

Set achievable goals:
Start by setting realistic and achievable goals for your exercise routine.
This can include a specific number of workouts per week, a target distance or duration for each workout, or a goal to increase strength or endurance.
Having a clear goal can help to motivate and guide your efforts.

Find activities that are enjoyable:
Choose activities that you enjoy, and that fit your interests and preferences.
This can help to make exercise more enjoyable and sustainable, and can reduce the risk of boredom or burnout.

Track progress:
Keep track of your workouts, and monitor your progress over time. This can help to keep you accountable, and can provide a sense of accomplishment and satisfaction as you see your efforts paying off.

Be consistent and persistent:

Stick to your exercise routine, and try to be
consistent and persistent.
Exercise can have long-term benefits, and
it is important to maintain a regular
routine to see results.

Don't give up:

If you face challenges or setbacks, don't give
up. Exercise can be challenging at times,
but it is important to keep trying and
to stay committed to your goals.
Remember the benefits of exercise, and
remind yourself of why you started
in the first place.

By following these tips, you can maintain a
regular exercise routine and reap the
maximum weight loss and health benefits.

Regular exercise is a valuable investment in your health and well-being. It can help to improve physical, mental, and emotional health, and can reduce the risk of chronic diseases.

Exercise can also enhance cognitive function, improve sleep, and boost mood. By sticking to a regular exercise routine, you can experience these benefits and improve your overall health and quality of life.

The effort and time that you invest in exercise will be worth it, and will pay off in the long run.

It is important to prioritize your health, and to make exercise a regular part of your routine.